DIY Hand Sanitizing Wipes for You

Step By Step Guide

Inex

responsibility of actions taken by the reader in conjunction with this work. The Publisher acknowledges that the reader acts of their own accord and releases the author and Publisher of any responsibility for the observance of tips, advice, counsel, strategies, and techniques that may be offered in this volume.

Table of Contents

Introduction

Congratulations on purchasing *DIY Hand Sanitizing Wipes for You,* and thank you for doing so.

In this day and age, you can't be too careful about germs. They linger just about everywhere—they are on the door handles that you touch, or the carts that you use to go grocery shopping. You can't know who or what has touched that surface beforehand. If you are out and about, it can be tough to even find paces that offer hand sanitizer, and sinks aren't always readily available. For these times, the best thing that you can do is make sure that you are using hand sanitizers or wipes. Of course, that requires you to be able to find them in the first place.

In this book, you will learn what you can do to begin to create sanitizers that can be used in several different forms. From being able to clean your hands effectively to making sure that you can ensure that the surfaces around you that you will be touching are sanitized. You need to trust that the sanitizers that you are using will work, and that means that you must make sure that you know what you are doing.

As you read through this book, you will learn all about what it will take for you to be able to create your own sanitizers at home. You will learn about what sanitizers do, how they work, and why it is imperative that when you do use them, they are measured out accordingly. You will be introduced to the most common and the most potent sanitizers that exist that can help you to keep yourself clean and ready to face whatever comes your way. Finally, you will be given several recipes that are designed to help you clean up—wipes, sprays, and gels. This means that you will have sanitizers for any occasion that you may need them and that you can take full advantage of knowing that when you need to be the cleanest, that you can be. When it comes to the matter of health and safety, not just for you, but for everyone, you can't take any chances, and that's why you have this book.

There are plenty of books on this subject on the market, thanks again for choosing this one! Every effort was made to ensure it is full of as much useful information as possible; please enjoy!

Chapter 1: How Sanitizer Works

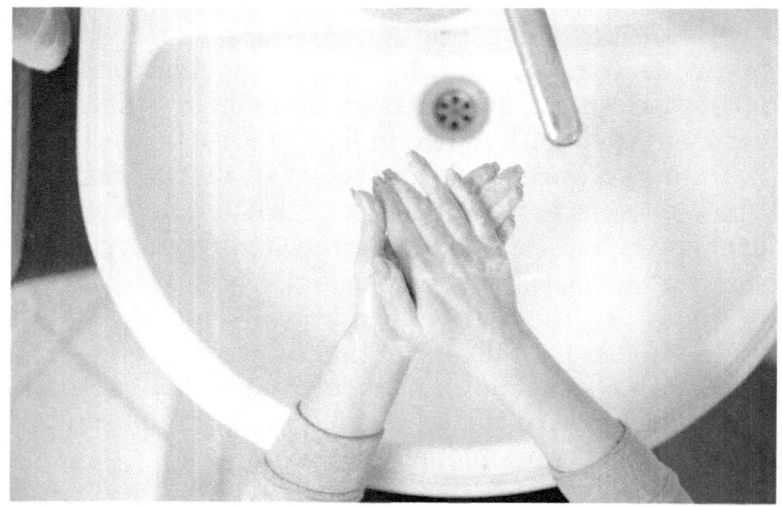

Before we begin, let's get one thing straight—hand sanitizer is not a replacement for handwashing. If you can do so safely and with the right equipment, washing your hands with soap and hot water is always the best method to ensure that you are keeping yourself clean enough to be safe. But, when you can't wash your hands safely, regardless of the reason, hand sanitizer is a decent second option.

Most hand sanitizers are made out of alcohol. This is what gives them their distinctive smell and the properties of evaporating shortly after use. Typically, they have around 70%, or sometimes more, alcohol content within them, and that alcohol is what kills the bacteria. While alcohol in moderation won't kill you, it is fatal to many viruses and bacteria. This is because the alcohol dissolves the outsides of the bacteria and viruses, meaning that their insides are no longer protected, and because of that, they die off quickly.

Many popular sanitizers tout that they are able to kill up to 99.999% of bacteria and viruses present on the body, and so many people think that it is the perfect substitute for washing hands—but the truth is, doing so actually isn't cleaning your hands. It may be killing off the germs, making it so that they can't reproduce or spread. However, while it does that, it does not remove the germs from the surface of the hand. Your hands are still going to be loaded up with the dead bodies of the germs that were on them. Sanitizer is effective at killing these germs, but it doesn't actually clean the hands. It simply sterilizes them.

This is why it is so important to use soap and water. When you do so, you are also getting all sorts of added benefits. You are making a point to ensure that your hands are actually clean—with soap and water, you are able to rub off the germs and wash them away like dirt. This is where the soap and water get their staying power—they may not kill off all of the germs, but they do remove them entirely, sending those germs flooding down the drain to be lost.

Because it only kills without removing the germs, you need to remember that ultimately, your hands aren't clean. You should still always go out of your way to find a source of water and soap to make sure that you can wash your hands. However, if you can't find a source, just keep it up with the hand sanitizer. While it may not remove the germs, it will kill them so that they can't infect you as well if you aren't careful. This means that you will be able to protect yourself and your family longer-term just by virtue of being aware of it.

Chapter 2: The Importance of Measurements

When you're ready to measure out your sanitizer, it is important for you to not that ultimately, the content of your sanitizer will vary based on the potency of the ingredients. Because of this, you must make sure that when you are making your sanitizer, you need to follow along and ensure that you not only meet all of the measurements that you are given, you also respect the ratios at which they are given and the concentrations that are requested. For example, if you are told to buy 70% alcohol and come back with 55%, do you think that it will be effective still?

Now, most people would say that of course it is still effective—alcohol is alcohol, right? The truth is, however, that that is not actually the case. The truth is that certain percentages of alcohol are more effective than others, and you need to have the right percentage if you hope to actually get some sort of sanitizing effect. Otherwise, people could just crack open a beer and use that to clean with—which wouldn't actually do much to help with cleanliness at all. When it comes to making sure that you choose out the right alcohol, you will need to ensure that it is strong enough, or the end product will not actually be effective. The effectiveness of it is entirely determined by the percentages of the product. Generally speaking, it is recommended that you have those larger ratios to ensure that you are properly getting enough alcohol to ensure that the sanitizer can work itself.

Whenever you are given measurements in this book, they are what they are for one specific reason— because those ratios are known to work. When you have that ratio written out, you know that the recipe has been created with the alcohol potency point in mind. If you start using different ratios, then you start to mess with the effectivity rate of those cleaners. If you are suddenly changing out how much of one ingredient that you are using, you will end up changing the potency. If you use 55% alcohol instead of 75%, you are already starting at a rate that is too low to be effective at all, and that means that you are creating a solution that is not actually going to be very beneficial to you in the first place. You will need to make sure that you take the time to actually use the proper ratios and concentrations, or you will create something that will not work. It is a science here, and that science depends on a very delicate balance that you must maintain. If you can't do that, you will struggle to create a proper sanitizer in the first place, and that means that you could be using something that is not going to actually kill the germs that you are attempting to avoid.

Keep in mind that, in this book, you can expect to see measurements that are designed specifically to allow for you to make the right potency that will help to ensure that you can properly sanitize surfaces. In particular, the magic ratio with sanitizers is that the alcohol must make up at least 60% of the content of your cleaner. If it does not hit that point, it has not been tested to ensure that it will work effectively, and that means that you can't know for sure just how well the sanitizer is working.

Remember that the recipes that you make on your own will not have been tested before. They should work if you have followed the instructions properly, but the truth is, unless you have made it a point to carefully measure each and every part of what you are doing, and you ensured that your ingredients were exactly what they were supposed to be, there is a chance that your sanitizer will not work. Remember that those industrial sanitizers that you can buy, or the commercially produced gels have to go through rigorous testing to ensure that they are FDA compliant as the over-the-counter products that they are classified as. However, your own sanitizers do not go through that process. You cannot assume that your sanitizers are going to work perfectly, though, and you should still always take the necessary precautions to ensure that you don't get sick. If you can make it a point to ensure that you aren't unintentionally making yourself ill, such as continuing to avoid touching your face after touching something and keeping your hands to yourself as much as possible, you should find that you are still much better protected than you would be without the sanitizer in the first place.

Chapter 3: The Most Common Sanitizing Ingredients

Now, you may be wondering which ingredients are going to offer you the best bang for your buck, and that is what this chapter here is for. As you read through this chapter, we are going to take some time to look at the most common sanitizing ingredients so that you know that you are able to properly prepare for the lists that you will see shortly. This chapter is here to provide you with how the most common sanitizing ingredients tend to work and what you can do to ensure that the ingredients that you are using will be effective. Generally, cleaning products are considered sanitizers if they remove 99.9% of germs present on something. Disinfecting agents must kill more than 99.999% in their entirety. Let's take a list at some that are highly capable of sanitizing and disinfecting surfaces now.

Isopropanol

Isopropanol is the primary chemical involved in rubbing alcohol and is the most commonly used disinfectant that you are going to see within this book. This is also commonly found in hand sanitizer thanks to its potency and ability to create effective disinfectants that generally aren't particularly harmful to humans. While it can be rough on the skin, especially if you don't usually make use of other ways to keep your skin softer, such as mixing it into aloe vera, you may run into a problem of causing skin irritation. It is recommended that if you use it on yourself, you do dilute it with something that will make it a bit gentler so that you aren't constantly worrying about the irritation.

Isopropanol is usually found listed as isopropyl alcohol in several different concentrations, typically between 50 and 99 percent. However, you will always want to choose the higher concentrations as those will allow you to know for certain that the alcohol is going to be effective. If you aren't careful, you can run into a situation in which you are using an alcohol that is too diluted and as a direct result, is not actually as effective as you think, putting yourself at extra risk.

However, keep in mind that these tend to lose their potency over time thanks to the fact that alcohol evaporates over time. It will effectively become less and less effective the longer that you have it. It is recommended that you don't store these containers of isopropyl for longer than a couple of years before it will have evaporated enough to begin losing its effectiveness.

Bleach

Bleach is another common disinfectant, but this one is far more caustic than the alcohol that you saw before. Bleach is effective because of the ingredient known as sodium hypochlorite—this is used to disinfect over time. When you make use of bleach, it is commonly used more as a surface cleaner than a skin cleaner. There are ways that you can create safe and effective hand cleaners with bleach, and this is commonly recommended by the World Health Organization in the absence of any sort of clean water source or running water that can be used. However, to be safe, the bleach must be diluted down significantly.

Bleach will burn the hands if you use it directly on your skin. It is irritating in nature, and if you will be handling it, it is highly recommended that you do so while making use of gloves to protect your hands as you do clean the various surfaces in your home. However, keep in mind as well that you must be mindful of what you mix into bleach. Certain ingredients, such as ammonia, are actually dangerous to mix into bleach, and if you try to do so, you will create toxic fumes that can be very harmful to your health. It is better to avoid this problem altogether and avoid it.

When you use bleach to sanitize surfaces, it is recommended that you apply it to the surfaces that you want to disinfect and then allow it to sit and air dry for a least 10 minutes. This gives it plenty of time to become effective, letting the bleach do its job to kill off whatever is on the surface. You will have to be mindful of what kinds of surfaces you use this with, as you can unintentionally discolor many fabric and soft surfaces that exist.

Hydrogen Peroxide

Hydrogen peroxide is also commonly used to clean surfaces as well—it is good to use to sanitize, though not usually as potent as bleach. However, it is shown to have disinfectant properties that will allow for it to kill viruses and bacteria, as reiterated by a 2018 study that found that hydrogen peroxide was quite effective at killing off certain bacteria. It is usually found and purchased at a 3% concentration rate, and you can purchase it just about anywhere.

It has been found to be effective against many common viruses, such as the ones that cause the common cold, and it is believed to be quite effective even just in the 3% concentration rate. You can use it directly, or you can cut it down to even 0.5%, at which point it would still retain some of the effectiveness. However, before you use hydrogen peroxide to disinfect, it is recommended that you usually make it a point to clean the area with soap and water first before adding the hydrogen peroxide right to the surface. Then, you must let it sit for at least a minute to let it get to work before taking the time to wipe it away.

While it is effective to use, you should not mix hydrogen peroxide with other cleaning agents unless specifically told to do so in the instructions for something. Likewise, you will want to make sure that you are mindful of the kinds of surfaces that you use it on. Certain countertops may be sensitive to the peroxide and end up with discoloration. It can also be irritating to your skin as well. It is best to wear gloves when working with the full 3% dilution rate, and you will also want to ensure that you make it a point to protect yourself.

Finally, keep in mind that hydrogen peroxide, if you are using it, reduces as it is exposed to light. It must be kept somewhere dark to make sure that it doesn't lose concentration, and therefore potentially also effectiveness.

Chapter 4: Are DIY Sanitizers Effective?

Now for the moment of truth—you are probably wondering if DIY hand sanitizers are even effective in the first place, and the good news is, yes, they can be. The catch is, however, that it is that they *can* be. This isn't a definitive yes, and the true answer is highly dependent upon the sanitizer that was created and how it was combined, stored, and used. However, there are a lot of criticisms that go into the idea of using a hand sanitizer or other form of sanitizer that was made at home without any real regard to potency or testing. This is mostly because we come from a culture in w which we must be mindful of what we use or endorse. We are a culture that is very sue-happy, and if something didn't work exactly as someone thought it would, there could be dire circumstances.

Sanitizers can be quite effective if you are able to get the right concentrations and ensure that they are mixed properly. This is the key here—a good sanitizer or disinfectant must have a proper disinfecting agent within them, and this means that you have to know what you are doing. However, if you can get it just right, you can be pretty confident (though never 100%) that you have something that will be just fine when you try to use it.

In order to be effective, your hand sanitizer or wipe will need to meet the following criteria:

- **Disinfecting agent:** Every effective solution must have some sort of agent that they can use to do the disinfecting for them. If you are able to choose out a disinfecting agent that you know will be effective, you are on your way to making sure that you will have an effective sanitizer.

- **Concentration:** It must have a rate of concentration that is acceptable and recommended to be capable of killing off pathogens in order to be effective. Not all concentrations that claim to be effective really are, so do your research to make sure that you are choosing one that will work.

- **Use:** Are you using your sanitizer the right way? This matters too—you can't just throw everything together and sort of just spritz off something before wiping it off immediately, only to say that it has been disinfected. The truth is, some of these must remain wet for several minutes in order to be fully effective. They won't just kill off bacteria and viruses in a few seconds of exposure. Give your sanitizer time to work.

- **Storage:** Likewise, if you don't store your hand sanitizer right, you run the risk of losing effectiveness as well. This happens because as you store it ineffectively, you will be degrading the ingredients. Alcohol evaporates, for example, so you can't just store your isopropyl, or your rubbing alcohol-based sanitizer in an open container without allowing the alcohol to just evaporate away. You must make sure that your ingredients and your sanitizer are both stored effectively so that you know that you won't be losing potency.

First, you must ensure that you have a disinfecting agent, which we discussed in the last chapter. The majority of the recipes that you will see to create your own sanitizers will rely on alcohol as it is one of the cheapest and most potent of the disinfectants that you can use. If you want to make sure that your sanitizer is effective, then you will want to make sure that it has some sort of disinfectant in it. Then, you must be mindful that the right amount is present, which is done by following the ratios. If you can guarantee that your solution has the right ratios and concentrations, you can be pretty confident that your cleaner will be potent enough to have the right effect on the surfaces on which it is used. You need to guarantee that you follow the recommended usage scenario, or you can't be certain that it will work either. Finally, you need to keep it all put away properly.

If you can go through each of those points and make sure that you are confident that your solution is created properly and stored properly, you can be pretty confident that it will be effective when it comes to cleaning your hands. Of course, there are no guarantees here—if you use these recipes, you are doing so at your own risk as these recipes are not regulated, nor are your own products ever tested by the FDA to ensure that they are actually as effective as they claim. Remember this—but realistically speaking, so long as you can get your ratios just right, you will probably be okay. That is a risk that you will have to take—however, some protection is better than no protection, and if you are caught between having to decide between using a homemade sanitizer or no sanitizer at all, your best bet is probably to use the homemade stuff.

Chapter 5: Using DIY Sanitizers

When it comes to using sanitizers, whether they are for your hands or for a surface, you must make sure that you are taking the necessary precautions to ensure that they are working effectively. This means that you must ensure that anything that you do is going to grant the right environment and set up for the sanitizer to do its job in the first place. Thankfully, using sanitizers is usually pretty self-explanatory once you know what you are doing and what to expect. You shouldn't run into any problems after reading over these different points to consider, and for that reason, you should commit all of these to memory before we begin. This way, you know that you are using the right types of sanitizers the right way. Consider these points, for example.

Gel on Hands

If you are using hand sanitizer on your hands, you must make sure that you first thoroughly coat your hands, and then you must continue to rub it until the sanitizer all evaporates. The evaporation tells you that the alcohol is doing its job, and that is how you are able to tell if it is working in the first place. Rub until the alcohol has all evaporated away.

Spray on Hands

This is used the same way—you want to thoroughly wet your hands with sanitizer and then allow it all to evaporate away over time. It will fade away, and you will know that you have allowed your hands to be cleaned.

Spray on Surfaces

If you are going to be spraying your sanitizer onto other surfaces, you know that you must cover the entire surface, and then you need to allow it to sit for a little while. Usually, it is recommended that you allow these sprays to sit for between 5 and 10 minutes to make sure that everything is truly neutralized on the surface, and then you are free to wipe it all away.

Wipes on Hands

If you are using hand sanitizer wipes on your own hands, you will want to first make sure that the wipe that you have chosen is hand-friendly. Some that are made for surfaces with bleach may be irritating and therefore are not recommended for hand use most of the time. Make sure that you are taking the time to wipe thoroughly, wetting your entire hand, and allowing them to linger.

Wipes on Surfaces

To use wipes on surfaces, you are going to want to ensure that you take the time to saturate the surface that you are using. This means that you will need to coat it with the liquid that is in your wipes, usually through making sure that you are constantly using fresh, moist wipes instead of trying to continue to make them work as soon as they are damp or starting to dry out. It is the liquid itself that is usually what does the disinfecting, so you will need to be mindful of that.

Chapter 6: DIY Hand Sanitizing Wipes

Wipes are a great option for cleaning on the go if you need to sanitize something that you are about to touch. For example, if you are going to the store, you may want to sanitize the handle of the shopping cart before you begin to use it. For this, you could try to use a gel or a spray, but either way, you will need a way to wipe over the surface, and that is oftentimes best done with a wipe.

The wipes that you could buy at the store are oftentimes expensive, and you don't get very many of them. However, if you want to make them yourself for easy storage, you have plenty of options available to you. You are able to make your own wipe recipes with ease if you know what you are doing. If you are going to be using wipes regularly, one of the greatest things that you can learn to do is to make them yourself, and this chapter will teach you to do exactly that. You will discover several options for doing so that will help you to ensure that ultimately, you can better keep your hands, your surfaces, and anything else clean.

As you go over this, one thing holds true—you are going to need paper towels and lots of them. These are going to be the most important part; if you are making disposable wipes, you need to be able to have a disposable material that you can use. From there, it is as simple as saturating those paper towels, which must be durable enough to endure the soaking in the first place, and then storing them for use.

If you are going to make your own wipes, it is recommended that you have some sort of waterproof, sealable container so that you can know that everything will stay moist. Containers that leak may allow for liquid to spill out, and that means no wetness for the wipes to do their job. You could consider using an old baby wipe box, or even the container from a pack of Clorox wipes. If you want some that you can take in your purse, there are plenty of diaper bag wipe containers that are small enough to take just enough wipes to need on one outing with a baby—those smaller portions are small enough to fit into a large purse or into a glove compartment in a car with ease if you chose to do so.

Now, let's start going over some great DIY recipes that you can use to create sanitizing wipes at home. These recipes will work great, so long as you know what you are doing, and so long as you follow the ratios that are given to you in this book! If you can remember that, you should have no problems with making your own with ease.

Basic DIY Wipes

This first recipe is something that you can make easily. It uses a simple mixture of alcohol, peroxide, some essential oils for scent, water, and something that you can use to hold your container together. Some people like to keep everything in a big jar while other people find that they prefer to make use of smaller containers that are sealable. That is entirely up to preference! You could even use a large plastic container with a lid on it if you choose—there is no rule to what your container has to be, so long as it can be sealed, and it will endure the saturation.

Ingredients

- A large jar or container to make your wipes in
- A roll of paper towels
- Essential oils of choice (up to 45 drops, only if you want your wipes to have a scent)
- Hydrogen peroxide (2 Tbsp. of 3% concentration)
- Isopropyl alcohol (2.25 cups of 99%)
- Water (10 Tbsp., purified)

To complete this recipe, all you have to do is get everything ready to go and combine it. It's really that simple—you'll be shocked that you never tried using these sooner! First, make sure that your paper towel rolls are the right size. There are many newer varieties of paper towels that tout that they are "choose your own size" rolls so that you can choose half-panels instead of whole squares, and those are highly recommended here to ensure that you have the flexibility to avoid using massive amounts at once. With these, you can simply take what you need—no more, no less.

You may also want to cut your paper towel roll down the middle to create two toilet paper-sized rolls, or even cut it into thirds if you don't want larger wipes. These are all great options—you just have to figure out which size you prefer. Simply take a serrated knife and cut where you want to.

Then, when your rolls are prepared, you can start mixing your sanitizer. In this case, you will combine your alcohol with the water and mix well, then add in the hydrogen peroxide and combine before finally adding in the essential oils. Mix them all well, and then move over to your jar. You will want to push your paper towel roll into the jar or container that you are using to store your wipes and then dump your sanitizer over the top.

After a while, the sanitizer should saturate everything, and you will be able to pull out the cardboard roll so that you can allow for the wipes themselves to be collapsed down for easier storage.

After a while, flip over the jar, with it sealed, so that the solution can get to all sides of the container and ensure that everything is well-coated. You can take a few out at a time and take them with you in a zippered plastic bag in a pinch.

DIY Hydrogen Peroxide and Alcohol Wipes

These wipes are a great option for you if you want to have some gently sanitizing wipes, especially because you can also choose to alter the recipe to be entirely peroxide-based if you don't want to deal with the alcohol, or if you find the alcohol to be too drying. This recipe is simple, smells great, and can be a great addition around your house to use or to use on your hands. They are gentle enough to be used either way but are tough on germs thanks to the peroxide and the alcohol.

Ingredients

- Baby wipe or Clorox container
- Essential oils of choice (30-50 drops to scent)
- Hydrogen peroxide (1.5 c, or 2 if you are going to omit the alcohol)
- Paper towel roll
- Rubbing alcohol (0.5 c., 190 proof)

To begin, prepare your paper towel roll. Cut it in half or thirds, as with the previous recipe, and then set it aside. Then, take a bowl and combine all of the listed ingredients until they are well-mixed. When you have combined it well, you can then put the paper towel roll into the container that you intend to use. Then, pour the liquid over the paper towels until thoroughly soaked and set aside to use later.

Disinfecting Wipes

This next recipe utilizes alcohol, water, and vinegar alongside soap to create a potent effect against all sorts of different germs that you may want to eliminate, and it is safe to use on your hands as well! No matter what you need them for, they are readily available and easy to use so that you can be certain that you are getting the best bang for your buck.

Ingredients

- Essential oil with scent of choice (10 drops)
- Filtered water (0.5 cups)
- Liquid soap (3 Tbsp.)
- Paper towel roll
- Rubbing alcohol (1 cup, 91%)
- Tea tree oil (20 drops)
- White vinegar (0.5 cups)

When you have all of your ingredients together, you are ready to begin creating the wipes. To begin, you must first cut the roll of paper towels in half or thirds. Then, you will want to take all of your liquids together, mixing them well. You should be able to do this in a bowl or cup without much of a problem. Make sure that they are all well combined.

Take your paper towel roll and put it into a jar so that you can properly push it into place. Then, drizzle the cleaning solution on top, soaking it. After a few minutes, you should be able to pull out the cardboard insert. Then, just make sure that the centermost paper towel is sticking up a bit so that you can pull them out and seal the container.

Alcohol, Tea Tree Oil, and Dish Soap Wipes

This next recipe is designed to work well if you want to clean your own home surfaces. The ratios are not quite right for straight sanitization, but that's because of the fact that you have dish soap added to them. The soap works to break down the coating on viruses to help the rest of the ingredients do their job while also deactivating the virus when the inside is damaged.

Ingredients

- Dawn dish soap (1 Tbsp.)
- Distilled water (1 cup)
- Isopropyl alcohol (2 cups, 90%)
- Paper towel roll
- Tea tree oil (3 drops)

To complete this recipe, all you have to do is get everything going and ready. Start by identifying where you are going to put your wipes—it is recommended that you use a large jar, as recommended earlier in this book. Then, prepare your paper towel rolls, cutting them in the middle or cutting them into thirds. Shove the paper towel rolls into the jars that you are using.

In a cup or bowl, combine your water, alcohol, soap, and oil and blend together well. You don't want to mix it so rapidly that bubbles form, but you do want the soap to have been diluted into everything. When the soap is well-incorporated, you can then add the liquid right into your jar, drizzling the liquid all over the paper towel roll. Don't just pour it all in at once—you may overfill your jar or container size. You also don't need your paper towels to be sitting completely submerged with lots of liquid left—you need there to be just enough that everything is thoroughly wetted. After a few minutes of soaking, remove the center of the paper towel roll, and seal the jar. After an hour, flip the jar upside down to redistribute any of the liquid that has settled at the bottom. Store it closed until ready to use.

Alcohol and Glycerin Wipes

This next container combines the cleaning power of alcohol with the moisturizing glycerin to ensure that your hands aren't going to dry out if you are using them too often. This is a great option to keep on hand to keep your hands clean. The wipes can also be scented with a few drops of essential oil if you prefer. This is entirely up to personal preference; however— you can choose to do this if you want to or forego it entirely. It is up to whatever you want.

The ingredients here are quite simple, and you can choose to either use a large airtight container or a large baggie to keep everything nice and moist so that when you need them the most, they will be available to you, even if you're not at home.

Ingredients

- Isopropyl alcohol (1.25 cups of 99%)
- Hydrogen peroxide (1 Tbsp.)
- Glycerin (1 tsp)
- Distilled water (0.25 cups)
- Paper towels (30, sliced in half

This recipe is quite simple to complete. Simply combine all of your wet ingredients until well incorporated. Then, when you have everything mixed well, put your paper towels into a baggie or a Tupperware container that you will be able to seal. Then, simply dump the mixture onto the paper towels, seal the container, and mix it well.

When you're ready to use these wipes, all you have to do is give the container a great shake before taking out the wipes that you will need. If your wipes are too saturated, give it a quick squeeze before wiping it all over your hands. Then, let your hands dry, and you're good to go.

Alcohol, Aloe Vera, Glycerin, and Oil Wipes

This next recipe packs a double moisturizing punch with both the glycerin and the aloe vera, meaning that it is quite gentle on the hands, even though it is able to sanitize well. If you find that you need to use gentler wipes because you have skin issues, such as eczema, this could be a great option for you so that you are able to keep your hands nice and healthy, even if you can't wash your hands as easily as you would like to. This is also gentle enough that your children's skin should tolerate it as well if you need to clean their hands as well.

Ingredients

- Alcohol (1.5 cups, 99% rubbing alcohol or 151-proof grain alcohol (Everclear)
- Aloe vera gel (2 ounces)
- Glycerin (2 tsp)
- Essential oils (1 tsp of choice to scent)
- Paper towels

Begin by combining your alcohol, glycerin, and aloe vera gel until it is well incorporated. It might be a bit thick, but that's okay. Then, combine in your essential oils as well to create the entire mixture. Then, put your paper towels into a container that you plan on using for storage. Pour your liquid concoction over it and seal, shaking well to combine.

When you use these, you will notice that they are wetter than usual—that's the gel, and it needs to be. Wipe the wipes over your hands and saturate your skin before letting it air dry.

Chapter 7: DIY Hand Sanitizing Sprays

While having wipes is a convenient option to have when cleaning your hands, it can also be somewhat wasteful to be using a single wipe every time that you need to disinfect something. Because of that, you may find that you are the happiest if you also have some sort of cleaning spray that will help you to avoid creating all of that extra waste. Having cleaning sprays can be just as convenient as wipes in many different contexts. A good cleaning spray is a great way for you to ensure that you are able to take your sanitizer with you without needing the extra bulk that is created by having the container as well. This means that you will be better prepared to clean surfaces without the paper towels, or you could even just carry around a bottle of spray in your pocket using a small perfume-sized bottle. There are many 2-ounce and 4-ounce spray bottles that you can take with you to use if you chose to do so, and those are great options if you want to avoid added bulk.

Within this chapter, we are going to look at some of the more effective recipes that you can find to create your own hand sanitizing sprays. If you prefer, you could also just take the solutions created in the previous chapter and use those as your spray without dumping them onto the paper towels. The solution itself should be potent enough to use. The recipes that you will find here can also be scented with different essential oils if you would prefer to have some extra smells to avoid smelling like you have just walked out of a doctor's office.

Consider all of these recipes to use. Some of them might work better for you than others, but all should be effective, granted that you take the time to follow the instructions and stick to the right ratios. They should help you to keep your hands clean and ready to go—all you have to do is make sure that you use them regularly!

70% Alcohol and Glycerin Spray

While only somewhat viscous, this option uses glycerin as a humectant, meaning that glycerin, a thick, syrupy substance, is used to keep your hands feeling soft. Despite the glycerin being added to thicken things up, this is another recipe that works well right into a spray bottle for easy use. This recipe is using 70% isopropyl alcohol and will create a sanitizer with roughly 63.5% alcohol within it, meaning that it is potent enough to keep your hands sanitized.

Ingredients

- 70% isopropyl alcohol (0.75 cups, plus 1 Tbsp.)
- Hydrogen peroxide (2 tsp, 3% concentration)
- Glycerin (1 tsp)
- Essential oils as desired for smell (up to 80 drops in the entire mixture)

Making this recipe is thankfully quite simple. All you have to do is take a jar, preferably roughly pint-sized, and with a lid for storage use. Put your alcohol and peroxide together, followed by the glycerin and oils of choice. Then, gently mix together everything until you can see that your glycerin has dissolved into everything. At that point, you have a potent spray that is going to be plenty effective once you put it into a spray bottle.

This makes enough for you to be able to fill up two small, 4-ounce spray bottles. It is highly recommended that you use a funnel for this process to avoid losing any of your mixture. Then, when it is done, you will want to let the bottles sit for at least 72 hours before using them. This is an extra precaution that you can use to ensure that your bottles are sanitary and that anything that may have been in the bottles beforehand has had a chance to be killed by the sanitizer.

To use this solution, all you have to do is give it a good shake, then provide a few generous spritzes to your hands, rubbing them thoroughly. Make sure that you don't spray the face or the eyes when you use it. This sanitizer will keep for around three months.

90% Isopropyl Alcohol and Glycerin Spray

This next recipe is markedly similar to the last one but is designed to be used with a higher concentration of alcohol—here; you are making use of a 90% alcohol spray. You'll notice that water is included on the list here, and you may think that's strange, but the truth is, the addition of water helps with the potency of the sanitizer.

Water helps by acting as a catalyst, the trigger that allows for the proteins of the membranes of the bacteria or viruses that you are going to kill. The water allows for the alcohol to penetrate better than if there were no water at all. Water also serves to slow down the evaporation speed of the alcohol, meaning that it will remain in contact with the microbes for longer. Science has shown that the higher percentages of alcohol, though effective, will require longer to be effective.

Ingredients

- 91% isopropyl alcohol (0.75 cups, plus 1 Tbsp.)
- Hydrogen peroxide (2 tsp, 3% concentration)
- Glycerin (1 tsp)
- Essential oils as desired for smell (up to 80 drops in the entire mixture)
- 4 tsp distilled water

Again, this is a very simple recipe—it is as easy as combining everything together into your jar and mixing well, just as with the previous one. You will still come out with about the same amount of fluid, and you should be able to use them the same way, splitting the mixture into two bottles and then allowing it to sit for 72 hours before using it.

Witch Hazel Spray

This next spray incorporates witch hazel, a commonly used astringent that has been traditionally used for centuries to aid in healing people. It is a powerful solution that is able to do great things for people, and it has been used medicinally for exactly that purpose.

It has been consumed to aid in the reduction of the flu or cold sores, but in this case, we are using it as part of our hand sanitizing spray. Of course, it is not the only ingredient that we are pulling into this for the destruction of any germs that we may have on our hands—we will also be bringing in rubbing alcohol as well. This recipe is not a very big one—you will notice that you will only get enough to fill a small, portable bottle—but you could scale it up if you wanted a larger container to take on the go.

Ingredients

- Witch hazel (2 Tbsp.)
- Tea tree oil (30 drops)
- Rubbing alcohol (3 Tbsp., 99%)
- Lavender essential oil (10 drops)
- Vitamin E oil (.25 tsp)

With all of your ingredients in mind, all you have to do is put them all right into a bowl or a cup. Make sure that you give it a good mix to make sure that everything is well incorporated and then add it into the bottle that you are going to use with a funnel. This

45

mixture is potent and smells great—you should be able to use it regularly thanks to the oil without your hands drying out as well! Just give it a good mix before you start to use it, spritz onto your hands liberally, and give it a good scrub, coating everything and preparing your skin.

Lemon Alcohol Spray

Though technically appropriate for hands if you wanted to use it, this is going to be best served as a disinfectant for objects rather than skin. This is because you don't have any sort of emollient to keep your skin nice and moist. However, in a pinch, it could be used if you didn't have anything else. This is a nice take on using alcohol to clean while still getting to enjoy a pleasant citrus scent. If you would prefer, however, you can make use essential oils instead of the lemons themselves.

This recipe will require you to leave it sitting for a while, but thanks to the small amount of ingredients that go into this one, you can use any alcohol that is above 60%, and you should get the effect that you are looking for. That means that if you have some 120-proof vodka or whiskey sitting around at home, you could use those for this purpose. Just keep in mind that if you are using alcohol from the store, you make sure that it is at least 120-proof, and make sure that it is also sugar- and additive-free. If it is flavored, it is going to cause problems with stickiness and residues.

Ingredients

- Alcohol (120-proof or above)
- Several lemons

And that's it—you don't even need to measure it out because you are not actually diluting anything! Fill up a jar with the peels of your lemons, making sure that the peels were cleaned beforehand, and then pour the alcohol into the jar. Fill it up near the top, seal up the jar, and then leave it to sit somewhere that is cool and dark so that your peels can begin to infuse with the alcohol. The scent is then infused right into the alcohol, much like how you are able to infuse alcohol with vanilla beans to create an extract.

Typically, you want to leave this sitting for at least six weeks if possible, but a bit less is okay if you don't want as strong of a smell. When you are done infusing the lemon skins, it is time to strain the liquid to ensure that it is nice and smooth. The easiest way to do this is to remove the peels and then pass the liquid through a cheesecloth or in a pinch, a paper coffee filter. The liquid should be a deep yellow color when it is ready. You can then put the liquid right into a spray bottle and use it to clean as many surfaces as you want.

If you choose to use this for hands as well, you should keep in mind that you will need to moisturize often, or your hands will get dry and peel.

Bleach Hand Washing Solution

This is a recipe that is used and recommended by the WHO for use when sinks or running water is not readily available. The only catch is that bleach evaporates rapidly—if you are using this to clean your hands, you will need to keep in mind that it is only really good for a single day before it gasses off to a point of no longer being effective. Because of that, you may find that it is not your favorite option.

As another note, bleach can cause problems on fabric or other surfaces as well, so you will need to be mindful of what you are doing and whether you are getting it onto things that it shouldn't be. This is being included in this book because it is a valid solution that you could use to spray and disinfect your hands, but you also have to be willing to recreate it. If you are going to be off the grid or camping for a while, this might be a great option for you to have, and it is better than having nothing at all.

Remember that this solution needs to be kept out of the reach of children and should not be considered for drinking either.

Ingredients

- Liquid bleach (2.6% chlorine)
- Water

To complete this recipe, you will need to know two distinct concentrations so that you can switch between them as necessary. There is a strong solution, which you can also use as a disinfectant if you need to clean surfaces and as a handwashing solution.

Strong solution

This solution is going to be irritating to the skin if you use it on yourself, so do not do so. Again, this is for cleaning surfaces, not people. This ratio is quite simple—it is just a 4:1 ratio of water and bleach. This means that you will add in 4 parts of water for every 1 part of bleach, mix well, and then use it. It can sanitize through soaking with 15 minutes.

Hand washing solution

To create the handwashing solution, you must take your strong solution and then dilute it down further to be at a concentration that your hands will be able to tolerate without being burned. This is achieved with a 9:1 ratio of water to strong solution. This means that for every 1 part of strong solution that you use, you must add in 9 parts water as well. You then use this cleanser to wash your hands just as you would if you were using soap and water—wet your hands and scrub well to ensure that you are cleaning all of the nooks and crannies and that you are ensuring that everything looks clean on your hands.

Chapter 8: DIY Hand Sanitizing Gels

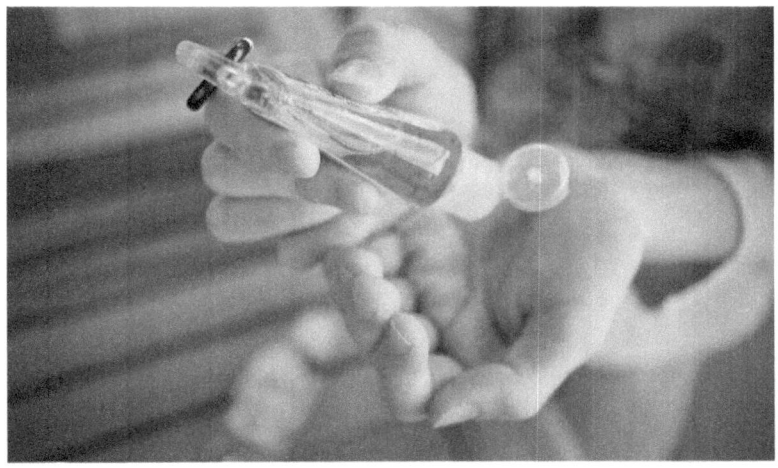

Now, we are going to take a look at several hand sanitizing gels that you can use that will help you to keep your own hands clean and sanitized when you need it the most. It's important when you are out and about, whether shopping, getting gas, or using an ATM, you are able to sanitize your hands quickly. If you touch something that is out in public, you need to be able to sanitize your hands to not only prevent yourself from getting sick but also so that you can prevent yourself from potentially spreading all sorts of germs all over the place as well. We know that every person has their own share of responsibility in making sure that they are able to help fight germs to keep them from spreading, and that means that you have to do your part as well!

Gels offer a convenient way for you to clean your hands without having to deal with a liquid that will just dribble away if you spritzed it, or deal with a wipe, which then creates something that you have to throw away. That means that with a gel, you can just take it on the go with you and squirt a bit wherever you need it.

We are going to look at a few different options for gels that can be sanitizing. As always, don't forget that the ratios of what you are making matters—you have to make sure that you are keeping the right concentration of sanitizing agent to everything else, or it is not going to be as effective.

Now, let's get started! These gels are easy to make, easy to use, and easy to take with you, too.

Isopropyl Alcohol and Aloe Gel

This is a simple enough cleaner to make and is perhaps the most common option that you will see online if you're looking for your own homemade recipe. This particular recipe blends together two common ingredients, creating a consistency that is quite similar to the commercial sanitizers that you are probably used to. However, keep in mind that aloe vera gel can leave behind a slightly sticky feeling on skin after it dries. That may be a small price to pay for having clean hands, however.

Make sure that your alcohol is the 99% variety, or it is not going to be as potent—this recipe is working with that particular ratio.

Ingredients

- Aloe vera gel (0.5 cups)
- Essential oils of choice (optional for scent—tea tree oil is common, but you can use lavender or other scents as well)
- Isopropyl alcohol (2 cups—99%)

This recipe is incredibly simple to complete. It's as simple as taking your alcohol and combining it right into your gel in a big bowl. It is important to do so in a bowl so that you can work well to emulsify it—making sure that there are no puddles of liquid or clumps of gel that have not been combined as that will hamper the effects of the cleaners.

When you have combined your liquid and your aloe vera gel, you can then add in a few drops of oils if you have chosen to add them. You don't need much—just a few quick droplets so that you can impart the scent to overpower the smell of sterile alcohol.

To store this particular sanitizer, you will find that a little squeeze bottle is the right way to go if you are taking it with you places. You can also use a pump bottle if you are keeping it in a larger quantity, such as if you are setting it next to your door to use as you come inside. All you have to do is use a funnel to help yourself put it right into the bottle without a mess.

If you notice that it starts to separate out, give it a good, thorough shake to blend it back together and use.

Everclear Alcohol, Aloe, and Witch Hazel Sanitizer Gel

If you find that you can't get your hands on isopropyl alcohol, the good news is that you're not out of luck! Certain alcohols for drinking do contain high enough concentrations of alcohol to use as a sanitizer, with the primary one that people think of being Everclear. This alcohol is banned in certain concentrations in certain states, so check for legalities before you set out to buy some. Everclear is incredibly potent, with some of them being at 190-proof, meaning that they are a massive 95% drinkable alcohol. Even the 151-proof, with a 75.5% alcohol content, can be difficult to find, depending on where you live.

This recipe recommends that you have the 190-proof Everclear, but if you don't, you could consider dropping down the rate of aloe vera gel down to 1/6 cup instead if you can get your hands on the 151-proof instead.

Ingredients

- Aloe vera gel (0.33 cup)
- Essential oil drops (up to 12 drops)
- Everclear 190-proof (0.66 cup)
- Witch hazel (1 ounce)

To complete this recipe is simple. It's literally just mixing together all of your ingredients and making sure that they are well-combined. You should get a loose, viscous gel as you do so. It is runny enough to pour, but not thick enough that you're going to have a hard time getting it out of a bottle.

This recipe can then be carefully scooped right into your squeeze container, or you can choose to put it into a pump bottle for use at home as well.

Conclusion

And that's that! We've made it to the end of this book, and you have now seen several different options for keeping your hands clean. They should all work in very similar ways, but the truth is, nothing is a better option than properly washing your hands with soap and water. There is a reason that using soap and water is the option of choice for doctors and surgeons around the world—it *works*. You need to remember that the options that you have been given in this book are designed to provide you with a quick clean if you need it—they will help you to ensure that if you are out and about and can't access a sink, you can still enjoy the protections of keeping your hands germ-free, but you should always opt for those other options when you have the chance to do so.

In this current world, we have to be more vigilant than ever—we are thinking about what we touch, what we touch after we touch that first thing, and more. We are starting to question just how dirty our hands are and how dirty the things that we touch are by extension. Remembering that we have to keep our own hands clean is an incredibly important point to remember that you will need to if you hope to be able to keep yourself safe and protected from any of the germs that are out there. No matter what it is that you are trying to avoid catching, making sure that you have the proper equipment is essential.

So, go out there. Be cautious as you enter the world around you and clean your hands often in any way that you can. If that means that you must clean them with some sanitizer, then do so. Enjoy life and make sure that you explore the world responsibly, doing your part to protect your community by making sure that you don't spread any germs further with careless touching.

Thank you for taking the time to get all the way to the end of this book! Hopefully, as you read, you found that it was incredibly helpful, and you have realized that you have several options for cleaning yourself up, even when you can't find a sink. If you've found that these different recipes have been helpful to you, please consider heading over to Amazon to leave a review! Your experience with these recipes is always greatly appreciated!